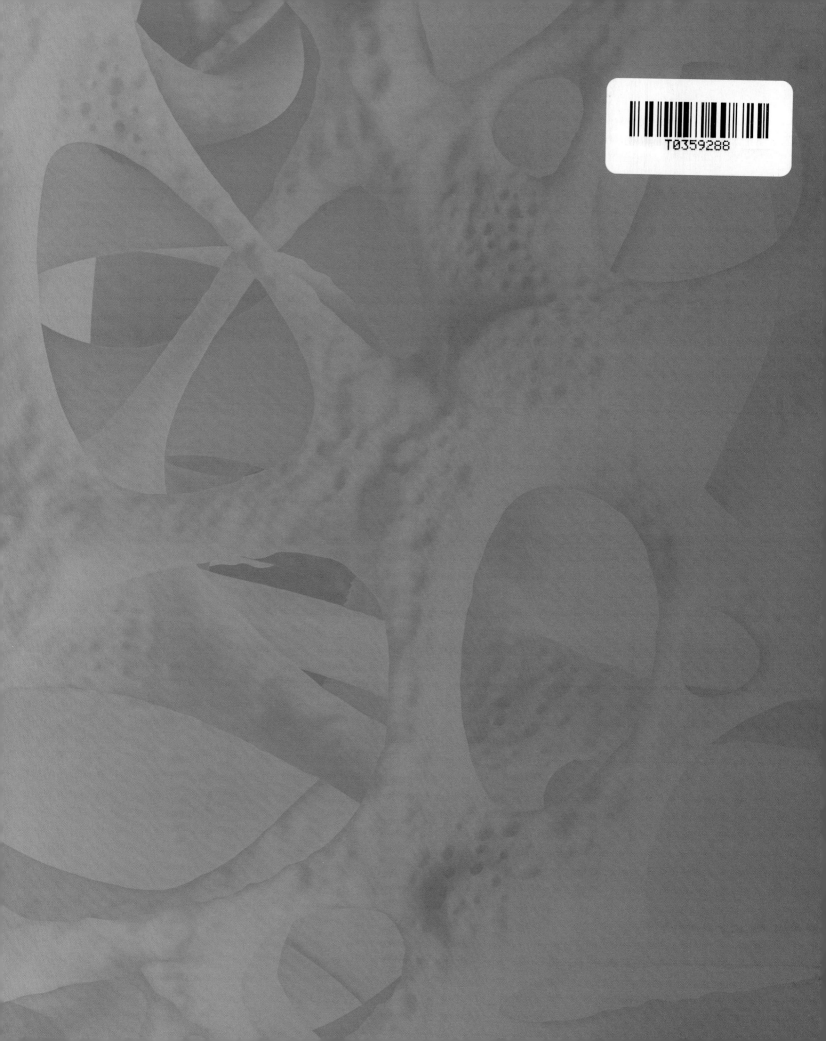

Australian GEOGRAPHIC

THE HUMAN BODY

How it works

THE HUMAN BODY

First published in 2021
Australian Geographic
52-54 Turner Street
Redfern NSW 2016
02 9136 7214

editorial@ausgeo.com.au
australiangeographic.com.au
© Australian Geographic
All rights reserved

Cover: solar22/Shutterstock (SS); Alex Mit/SS; Anatomy Image/SS; decade3d - anatomy online/SS; Anatomy Image/SS; itsmejust/SS; eranicle/SS; Anatomy Image/SS.
Contents: AridOcean/SS.
Glossary: i9yiyiXV/SS.
Back Cover: Puwadol Jaturawutthichai/SS.

Creative director: Mike Ellott
Designer: Harmony Southern
Editors: Lauren Smith and Peter Tuskan
Print production: Katrina O'Brien

Australian Geographic
Managing Director: Jo Runciman
Editor-in-Chief: Chrissie Goldrick

The Australian Geographic Society was established to encourage the spirit of discovery and adventure, and to foster love for our natural heritage. The Society and the Australian Geographic journal sponsor scientific research and conservation, and a portion of the profits from our published products goes back into the Society. Become a member today by subscribing to the Australian Geographic journal.

Subscribe now: 1300 555 176 or australiangeographic.com.au

Printed in China by Leo Paper Products Ltd.

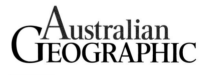

NATIONAL LIBRARY OF AUSTRALIA

A catalogue record for this book is available from the National Library of Australia

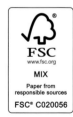

FSC
www.fsc.org
MIX
Paper from responsible sources
FSC® C020056

CONTENTS

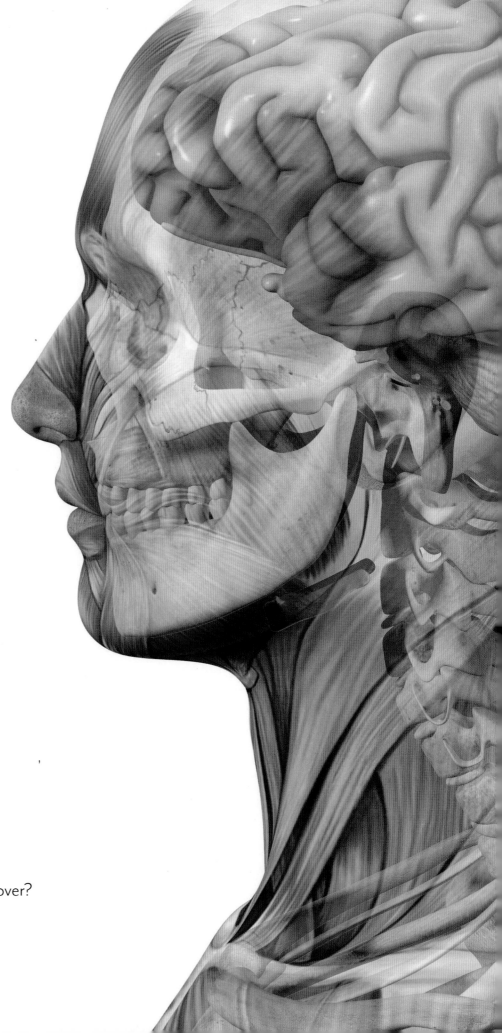

WHAT IS THE BODY MADE OF?

It's more than just blood and bones.

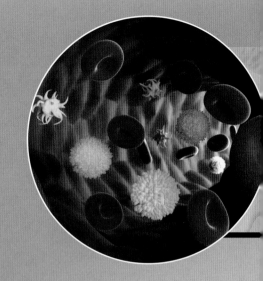

The human body is an incredible feat of nature. It works in very complicated ways so that we can experience life.

If you zoomed right in to see the body's most basic parts, you'll find atoms – the building blocks of life. Atoms are so small that about 7,000,000,000,000,000,000,000,000,000,000 (7 octillion) fit inside the body of an adult.

Different atoms make up different elements. Your body is mostly composed of four elements: oxygen, carbon, hydrogen and nitrogen. They make up 96 per cent of your body. Oxygen and hydrogen are the two elements found in water, and your body is about 60 per cent water. Carbon is the essential element for life – the key ingredient for all living things on Earth. Carbon is a necessary part of the **proteins**, **carbohydrates** and fats that make up the human body.

Nitrogen is found in many places in your body, including the acids that make up proteins and DNA. Many other elements are also found throughout your body.

Atoms combine in molecules, which group together as cells. Cells, grouped together, make up different components of your body, including your muscles, bones and organs.

These components connect in a variety of systems in your body that allow you to breathe, that pump blood around your body and that keep you functioning and healthy. These complex systems, such as the respiratory system, involve whole chains of intricate machinery such as your lungs, your diaphragm and your mouth.

These systems work together to allow you to do things like eat, drink, run, walk, dance and laugh.

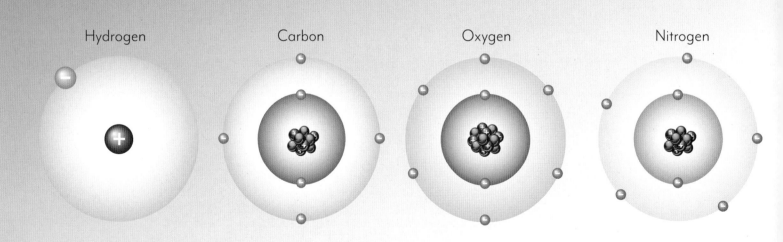

Hydrogen   Carbon   Oxygen   Nitrogen

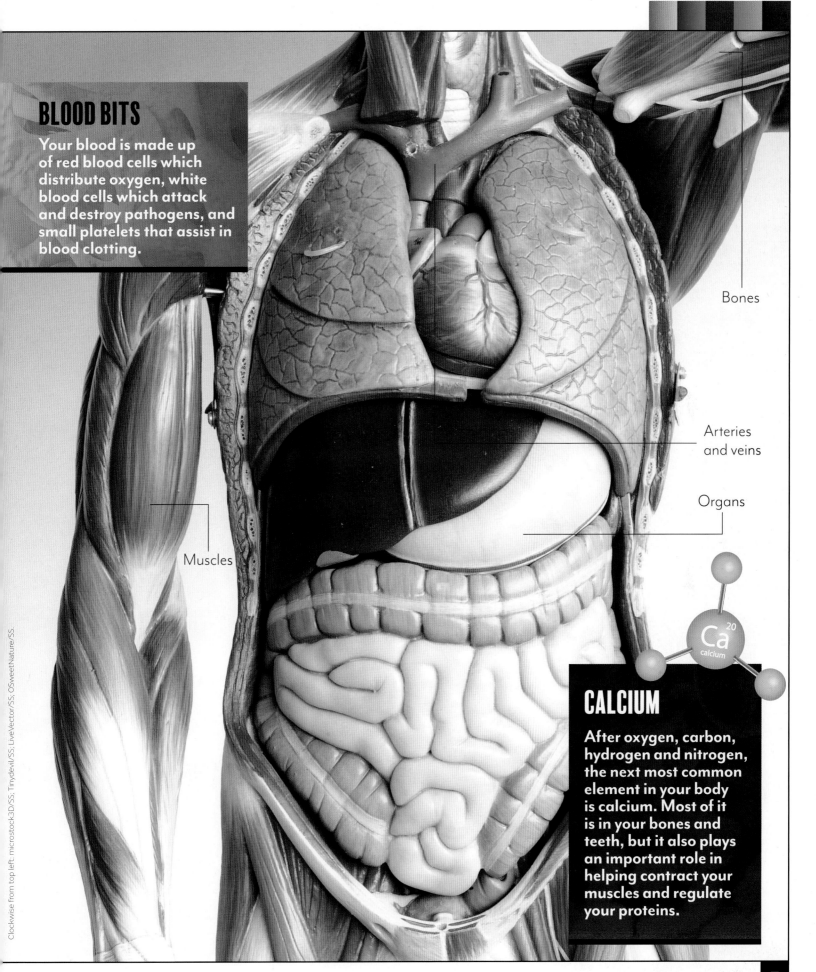

BLOOD BITS

Your blood is made up of red blood cells which distribute oxygen, white blood cells which attack and destroy pathogens, and small platelets that assist in blood clotting.

Bones

Arteries and veins

Organs

Muscles

CALCIUM

After oxygen, carbon, hydrogen and nitrogen, the next most common element in your body is calcium. Most of it is in your bones and teeth, but it also plays an important role in helping contract your muscles and regulate your proteins.

HOW DOES THE BRAIN WORK?

Your brain is the control room for your body.

Your **character and** personality are determined by your brain. All of your thoughts, ideas and emotions come from here. Scientists are still learning about the brain, as it's an incredibly complex organ. Let's look closer at the different parts of the brain and see what they do.

The right side of your brain controls the left side of your body. This side is also responsible for making sense of visual and **auditory** cues, facial recognition and 3D **spatial** awareness. The left side of your brain is responsible for the right side of your body, and also handles your language and verbal skills, as well as logical processing – like dealing with a maths problem.

The outer, folded layer of the brain is called the cerebral cortex. It's broken up into four areas: the temporal, occipital, parietal and frontal lobe.

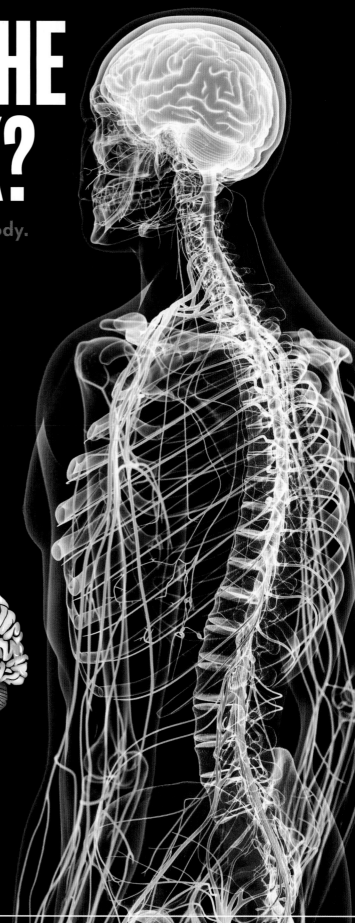

The brain is not only the source of our ◆ personality and the overseer of our body, but it's also the main organ that controls our nervous system.

DIFFERENT PARTS OF THE BRAIN

1 The **frontal lobe** is where your personality and character stem from. It's also responsible for memory, making decisions, generating ideas, social behaviour and problem solving.

2 The **anterior cingulate gyrus** monitors elements of the cardiovascular system, looking after your heart rate and blood pressure. It's also involved in some **cognitive** functions, like empathy and decision-making.

3 The **parietal lobe** processes nervous signals to do with your sense of taste, temperature and touch.

4 The **occipital lobe** is your brain's vision centre – it's where what you see gets processed into information. It's also responsible for generating the dreams you have at night.

5 The **temporal lobe** is the audio centre, where hearing and speech is managed. This lobe also handles memorisation of faces and signs.

6 The **hypothalamus** is part of your hormonal system, monitoring temperature, hunger, thirst and tiredness.

7 The **hippocampus** is where all of your memories are stored.

8 The **amygdala** is responsible for generating fear.

9 The **thalamus** is where all of the signals from your nervous system first arrive. From here, those sense signals are sent out to the brain to be processed.

10 The **cerebellum** coordinates your motion. It's integral for balancing, walking and more complicated activities like riding a bike.

SKELETAL SYSTEM

— Cranium

FUNCTION: Movement, protection and storage

MAIN STRUCTURES: Bones and tendons

WORKS CLOSELY WITH: The muscular and cardiovascular systems

MEDICAL FIELD: Orthopaedics ("or-tho-pee-diks")

Clavicle

Scapula —

Humerus —

Spine

— Ulna

Pelvic— girdle

Sacrum

— Femur

Patella

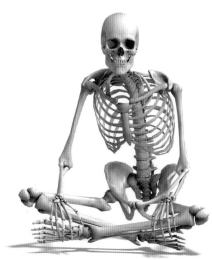

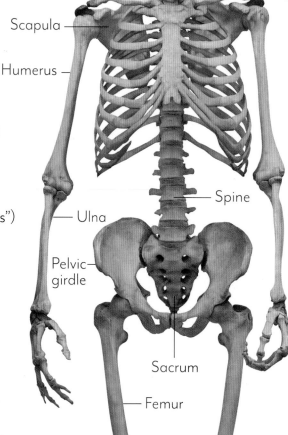

Tibia —

Fibula —

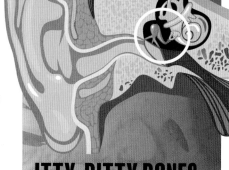

ITTY-BITTY BONES

The smallest bones in your body are inside your ear. There are three tiny bones – the hammer, the anvil and the stirrup – and all three help us to hear!

The skeleton supports the body and gives it shape. Bones contain living tissues with a blood supply and change shape over a lifetime. Bone tissue contains three types of cells. Osteoblasts make new bones and help to repair damage. They mature into osteocytes, which continue to produce new bone cells. Osteoclasts break down bone and are responsible for shaping bones. These all help our bones to grow, and aid in healing if they should be broken. Newborn babies have around 300 bones, but adults only have 206, because some of our bones fuse together as we age.

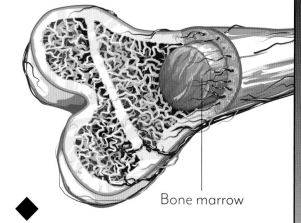

Bone marrow

◆

Inside our bones is a material called bone marrow, and it produces our blood cells – up to 500 billion every day!

MUSCULAR SYSTEM

FUNCTION: Movement, strength, balance, heat

MAIN STRUCTURES: Muscles and **fascia**

WORKS CLOSELY WITH: The skeletal and cardiovascular systems

MEDICAL FIELD: Physiotherapy ("fiz-ee-o-ther-a-pee")

Trapezius

Deltoid

Bicep

Brachioradialis

Finger flexors

Abdominals

Quadriceps femoris

Gluteus maximus

Tibialis anterior

Achilles tendon

Together with the skeletal system, muscles allow us to move about. There are three types of muscles. Smooth muscles, such as the bladder and stomach, are involuntary ones. We don't have any control over them, but they perform vital tasks such as moving food through the digestive system. The cardiac muscle, the heart, is a special involuntary muscle that modulates its beating to send the right amount of oxygen and blood around your body. Skeletal muscles are voluntary ones, which we're in charge of. These are attached to the skeleton by tendons. When you contract a muscle, it tugs on tendons, moving your bones.

◆

You have more than 640 muscles in your body, making up more than half of your weight.

MAGIC MOVERS

Pulses from the nervous system trigger the fibrous strands of your muscle, forcing them to contract. Muscles are the only tissues in your body that have the ability to contract and cause movement.

HOW DO THE SENSES WORK?

Most people have five senses: touch, taste, smell, hearing and sight.

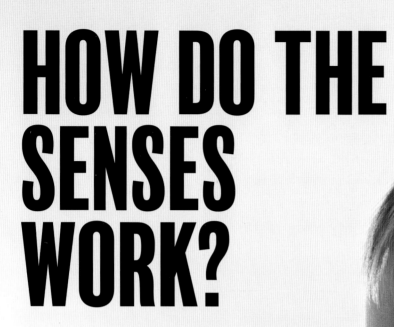

Senses are what allow you to understand the world around you. Thanks to them, you can smell flowers, touch your toes, hear your favourite song, see the sunset, and taste delicious foods. These five senses each work with a sensory organ; your nose, skin, ears, eyes or mouth. Not only do they allow you to experience good things, but they can also warn you about dangers, such as touching a hot stove or smelling smoke. The sensory organs contain receptors that communicate the information they receive with your brain via the nervous system. For some people, these senses may be lessened or completely gone – these people may be deaf or blind, for instance.

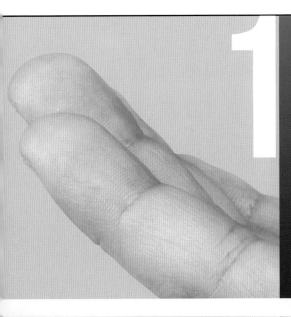

1 TOUCH

Touch is the sensation you get when nerve receptors in your skin come into contact with something else. The receptors send signals via the nervous system to the part of the brain responsible for the area where the sensation was felt. They tell the brain information about how and what you're touching, such as whether it's hot, cold, soft, or hard, and whether you're touching it softly or strongly.

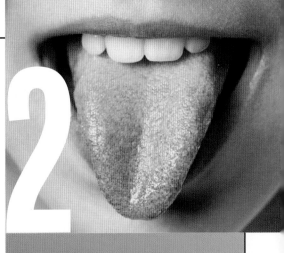

2 TASTE

Did you know you can sense five basic tastes: sweet, bitter, salty, sour and umami? When you eat ice-cream, little taste buds on the top of your tongue sense that it's a sweet food and send that message to your brain. If you put something yucky in your mouth, your taste buds will identify it as tasting bad, and your natural reaction will be to spit it out.

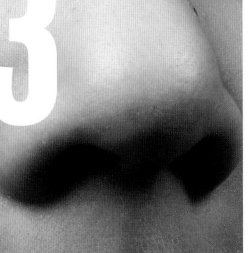
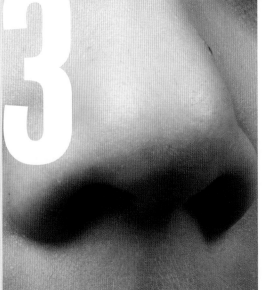

3 SMELL

Smell and taste work closely together, which is why sometimes you can't taste anything when you have a blocked nose. Airborne particles enter your nose through your nostrils and from the back of your mouth. These particles stimulate your **olfactory** receptors, which then communicate with your brain via the olfactory nerve. The more olfactory receptors a creature has, the better it can smell. Humans have about 15 million olfactory sensors. Some dogs have about 4 billion, which allows them to smell much better than us!

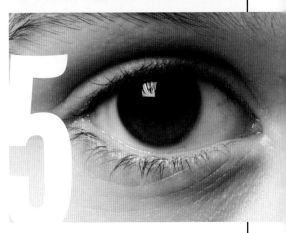

5 SIGHT

Your eyes allow you to build a picture of the world around you. Your eyes detect visible light and focus it on the retina, a section at the back of the eyeball. There are millions of light-sensitive cells on your retina, called rods and cones. They convert light into electrical signals that are then sent to your brain along the optic nerve. The brain's job is to interpret those signals so you can recognise and understand what you're seeing.

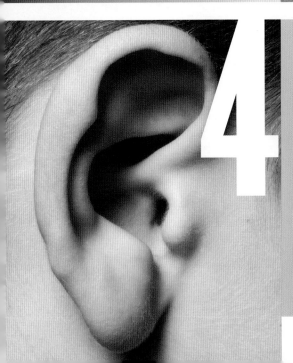
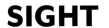

4 HEARING

Soundwaves hit your eardrum, a tightly stretched piece of skin, causing it to vibrate. These vibrations pass along the bones in your middle ear called the hammer, stirrup and anvil, or collectively, the 'ossicles'. The ossicles transfer the vibrations into your fluid-filled middle ear, or cochlea, creating waves. The waves move tiny hairs, and when the hairs realise they're moving, they send chemical signals to the auditory nerve, so your brain can interpret the vibrations as sound.

CARDIOVASCULAR SYSTEM

FUNCTION: Transportation of nutrients, waste and hormones

MAIN STRUCTURES:
The heart and blood vessels

WORKS CLOSELY WITH:
The immune system

MEDICAL FIELD:
Cardiology ("car-dee-olo-gee")

With each beat, the heart pushes blood around the body, bringing oxygen and nutrients to the cells. When we breathe in oxygen, it is absorbed into our blood through our lungs. The heart pumps this oxygen-rich blood through arteries until it reaches the organs, muscles and nerves. Here, it moves into tiny capillaries, through which the cells can absorb the oxygen. The blood then flows through veins back to the heart and lungs so it can collect more oxygen and start the cycle again.

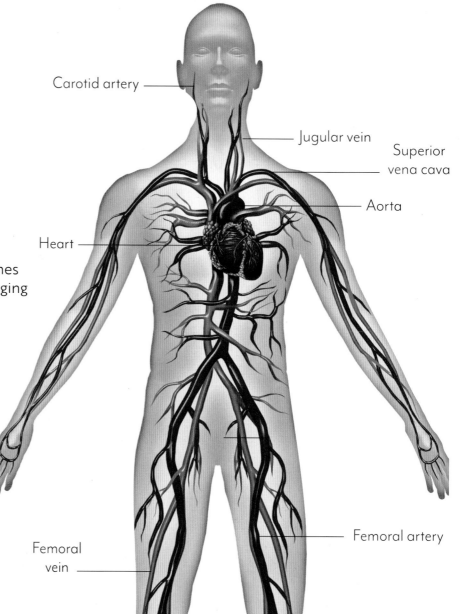

Carotid artery

Jugular vein

Superior vena cava

Aorta

Heart

Femoral artery

Femoral vein

BLOOD TYPES

There are different types of blood, determined by the type of red blood cells you have. The main blood groups are O, A, B and AB, though 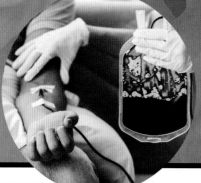 there are minor variants of these groups. If you ever need a **transfusion**, the doctors will need to check what blood type you are to make sure you receive a compatible type of blood.

NERVOUS SYSTEM

FUNCTION: Reactions, senses and digestion

MAIN STRUCTURES:
Brain, spinal cord and nerve cells (neurons)

WORKS CLOSELY WITH:
The integumentary system

MEDICAL FIELD:
Neurology ("newr-ol-o-gee")

If you feel pins and needles, it's because you've accidentally squished a fascicle, which is a bundle of blood vessels and nerves.

The nervous system controls both our voluntary and involuntary actions. It uses electrical and chemical signals to help different parts of the body communicate with each other. The signals travel along a highway made up of neurons. The neurons connect, dendrites to axon terminals, to make nerves. If you stand on something sharp, a sensory nerve in your foot will send a signal to your spinal cord, telling it to move. Simultaneously, the sensory nerve will signal to a motor nerve to stabilise the other side of the body, and to contract the necessary muscles so that you can maintain your balance. All of these messages pass through your brain. This all happens in less than a second. The nervous system is also responsible for telling the heart to beat, the lungs to pump and the stomach to digest, among other things. This is known as the autonomic nervous system.

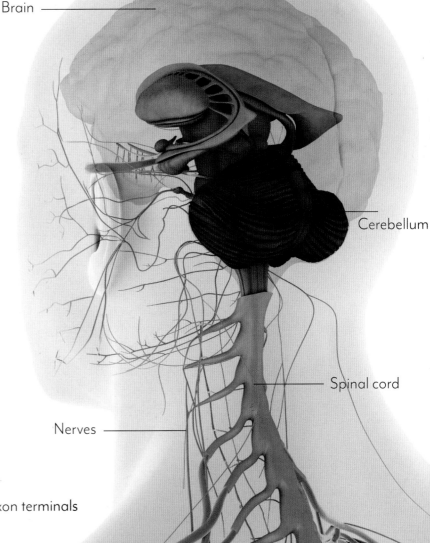

Brain

Cerebellum

Spinal cord

Nerves

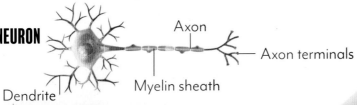

NEURON

Axon

Axon terminals

Myelin sheath

Dendrite

WHY DO HUMANS NEED SLEEP?

We're asleep for about one-third of our lives, but have you ever wondered why?

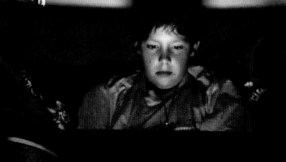

When you get tired, you know that it's time for bed. When you wake up from a full night of sleep, you feel more alert, more energetic and happier.

When you don't get enough sleep, it hugely impacts you. You'll have reduced alertness and memory, a shorter attention span, slower reaction times, poorer judgement and an increased chance of being angry or grumpy. If you're deprived of sleep for a long time, it can increase your risk of serious ailments such as heart disease, diabetes, obesity and depression.

When you do sleep well, science has shown that your muscles grow, your tissues repair themselves and certain hormones are released. It's an opportunity for your body to grow and repair itself. It's also important for development. Newborns sleep for up to 17 hours a day, and the amount you need to sleep slowly decreases until you're an adult. By this stage, your body needs between seven and nine hours a night. A recent theory suggests that sleep plays a role in the shaping of memories, which helps us to learn new information.

SLEEP-WAKE CYCLE

Your SCN (suprachiasmatic nucleus), which is your body's clock, perceives light and sends messages to the body and other parts of the brain about what processes should be taking place.

The pineal gland in your brain uses that information to determine how much melatonin to produce. Melatonin is a hormone that aids in regulating your day-night sleep cycle, also known as your circadian rhythm.

Your eye perceives light and sends a message to your brain about how much light it senses.

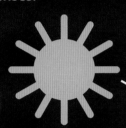

More melatonin is sent out as the light dims, hastening the onset of sleep.

The message passes through the SCG (superior cervical ganglion), an important part of your nervous system, and then up to the pineal gland.

WIDE AWAKE

The longest recorded period that someone intentionally went without sleep was more than 18 days. The participant said that he experienced paranoia, memory lapses, hallucinations and blurred vision.

HOW MUCH SLEEP DO YOU NEED?

0–3 months	4–24 months	3–5 years	6-13 years	14–18 years	19–65 years	66–90 years
14–17 hours	12–15 hours	10-13 hours	9–11 hours	8–10 hours	7–9 hours	7–8 hours

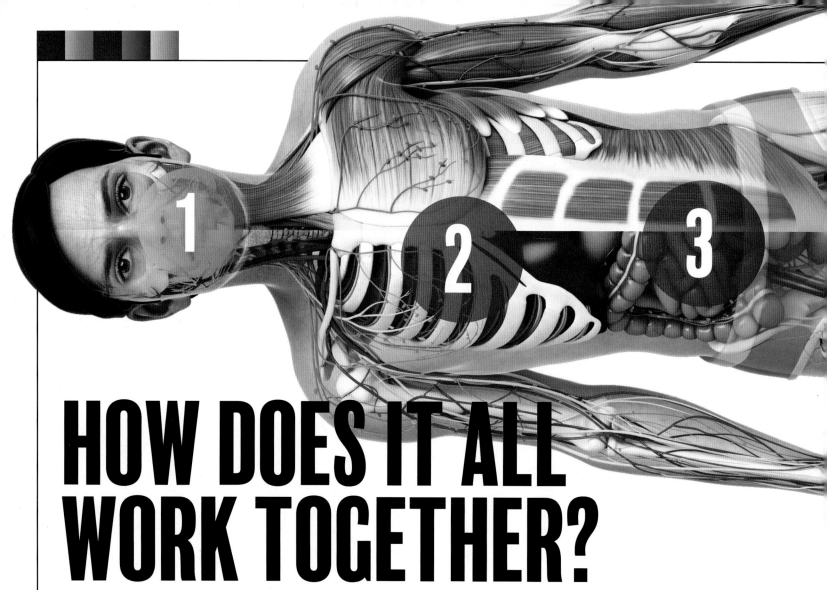

HOW DOES IT ALL WORK TOGETHER?

Our different systems and processes work in harmony to keep us going.

1 If you breathe in something bad, such as a germ, your immune system often will recognise it and send a message to your brain that the invader doesn't belong. Your muscular and skeletal system work together to create contractions that lead to coughing, hopefully ejecting the **pathogen**.

2 The cardiovascular and respiratory systems work closely together. The central organ of the cardiovascular system is the heart, and it pumps blood that the kidney has just cleaned straight into your lungs, where the respiratory system re-oxygenates it through the alveoli.

S K Chavan/SS; Carolyn Frank/SS; LightField Studios/SS; Maxim Khytra/SS; martan/SS; Luis Molinero/SS.

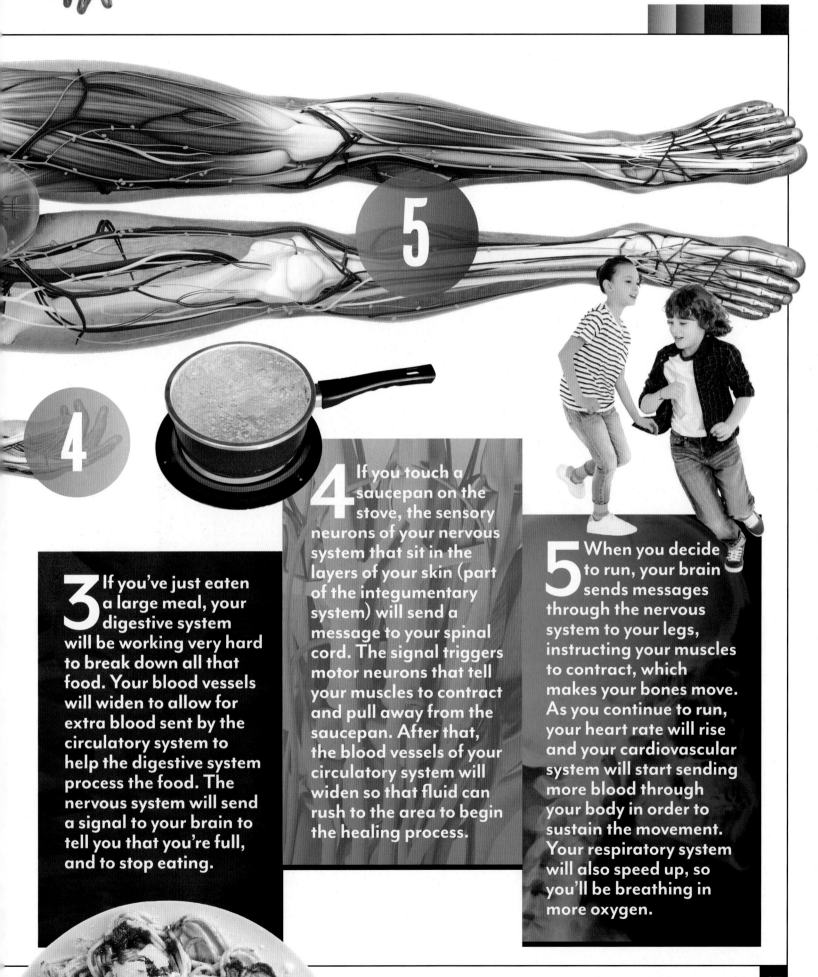

3 If you've just eaten a large meal, your digestive system will be working very hard to break down all that food. Your blood vessels will widen to allow for extra blood sent by the circulatory system to help the digestive system process the food. The nervous system will send a signal to your brain to tell you that you're full, and to stop eating.

4 If you touch a saucepan on the stove, the sensory neurons of your nervous system that sit in the layers of your skin (part of the integumentary system) will send a message to your spinal cord. The signal triggers motor neurons that tell your muscles to contract and pull away from the saucepan. After that, the blood vessels of your circulatory system will widen so that fluid can rush to the area to begin the healing process.

5 When you decide to run, your brain sends messages through the nervous system to your legs, instructing your muscles to contract, which makes your bones move. As you continue to run, your heart rate will rise and your cardiovascular system will start sending more blood through your body in order to sustain the movement. Your respiratory system will also speed up, so you'll be breathing in more oxygen.

RESPIRATORY SYSTEM

Breathing is so vital to our survival that our bodies do it without us having to think about it. Every time we breathe in, we are inhaling oxygen (O_2) into our lungs. Without oxygen, the cells in our bodies would die. The oxygen we inhale travels to the cells in the bloodstream. It gets into the bloodstream through tiny air sacs in the lungs called alveoli, which have very thin walls that oxygen can pass through. When you inhale, the diaphragm (a thin sheet of muscle below your lungs) contracts and the muscles in the chest lift the ribs up. This creates more space in the lungs for air, and they fill up like balloons. We inhale about half a litre of air with every breath we take.

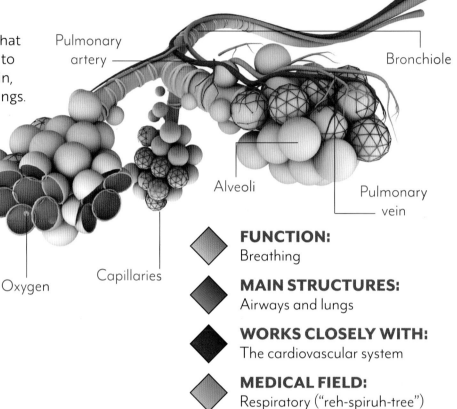

Pulmonary artery

Bronchiole

Alveoli

Pulmonary vein

Oxygen

Capillaries

◆ **FUNCTION:**
Breathing

◆ **MAIN STRUCTURES:**
Airways and lungs

◆ **WORKS CLOSELY WITH:**
The cardiovascular system

◆ **MEDICAL FIELD:**
Respiratory ("reh-spiruh-tree")

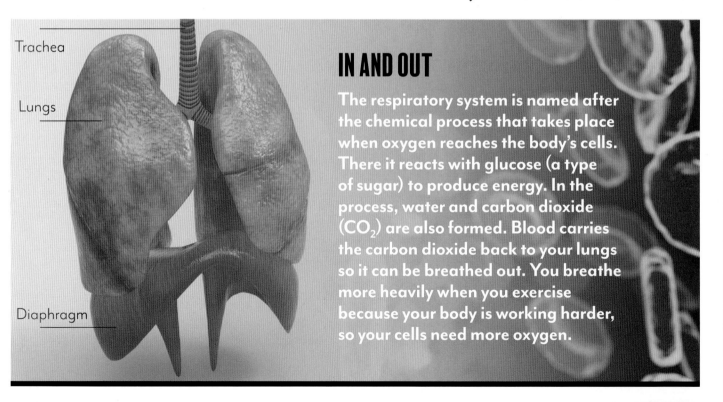

Trachea

Lungs

Diaphragm

IN AND OUT

The respiratory system is named after the chemical process that takes place when oxygen reaches the body's cells. There it reacts with glucose (a type of sugar) to produce energy. In the process, water and carbon dioxide (CO_2) are also formed. Blood carries the carbon dioxide back to your lungs so it can be breathed out. You breathe more heavily when you exercise because your body is working harder, so your cells need more oxygen.

DIGESTIVE SYSTEM

FUNCTION: Absorbs nutrients from food and removes waste

MAIN STRUCTURES: Mouth, stomach, intestines and liver

WORKS CLOSELY WITH: The immune system

MEDICAL FIELD: Gastroenterology ("gas-tro-enter-olo-gee")

The liver is the largest internal organ in the body. It performs about 500 different functions.

The digestive system breaks food down into very small pieces so nutrients – including carbohydrates, proteins and fats – can be absorbed into the bloodstream. Food travels from the mouth through the throat and into the oesophagus. It then goes down into the stomach and is broken up by stomach acids before moving into the small intestine, where it can stay for hours. The small intestine, which can be up to 7m long, is where most of the nutrients from our food are absorbed. **Villi** (tiny worm-like structures) stick out, collecting nutrients to pass into the bloodstream. After that, the leftovers are pushed into the large intestine (or colon), which can take about 12 hours to process food. Anything left at the end leaves the body as faeces, or poo, through the rectum.

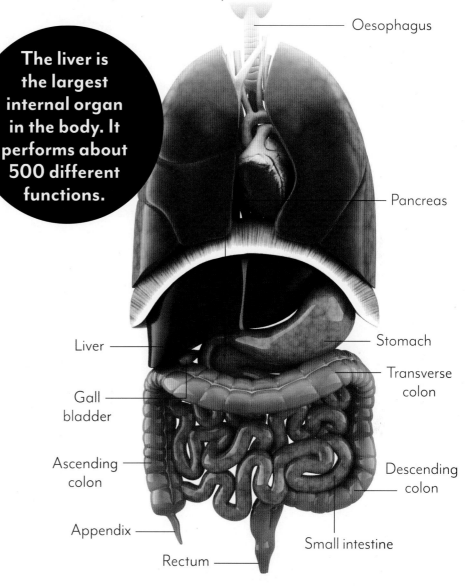

Oesophagus

Pancreas

Liver

Gall bladder

Ascending colon

Appendix

Rectum

Stomach

Transverse colon

Descending colon

Small intestine

BUSY BODIES

The pancreas produces digestive **enzymes** and releases insulin into the bloodstream, which helps to manage sugar levels. The liver produces bile, which is stored in the gall bladder and then pumped into the intestines to help break down food. The liver also filters all of our blood, making sure that anything harmful doesn't continue to travel through the body.

HOW DO HUMAN BODIES FORM?

Humans have a reproductive system for making babies. Men produce sperm and women produce ova.

Ovum

Sperm

When these two cells are united in the female womb, the egg (ova) is fertilised and begins to grow into a baby. The fertilised egg will divide itself over and over, continually doubling and growing. Over the next nine months, that single cell will grow into a baby made up of five trillion cells.

THE FIRST WEEK

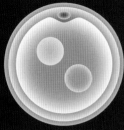

Zygote formation (24 hours)

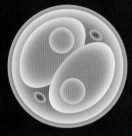

Two cell stage (36 hours)

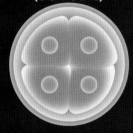

Four cell stage (48 hours)

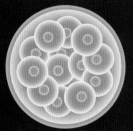

Morula (4–5 days)

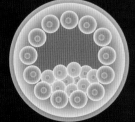

Blastocyst (6 days)

When the embryo has divided enough times to make a clump of 32 cells, it is called the morula stage. If the embryo has split at some point before then, it can grow into identical twins.

By six days old, the **embryo** consists of only a few hundred cells. Some cells will be part of the developing embryo, and others will be part of the placenta (the protective organ that surrounds, protects and nourishes the embryo).

At three weeks, the embryo still doesn't look very human, but the cells will be specialised – cells for the skin, brain and nerves; cells for the muscles, vessels, bones and certain organs; and cells for the gut, stomach and lungs. After this point, the embryo starts to shape the body. Between four and eight weeks, limbs and organs will start to grow.

At about nine weeks, the fetus, or baby, has started to develop clearly human features such as limbs. It is connected to the mother by the umbilical cord, which is how it receives oxygen and nourishment.

Biological females have 23 pairs of X chromosomes, like this one, in their genes. Biological males have 23 pairs made up of an X and also a Y chromosome.

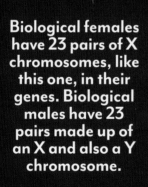

HUMAN BODY MANUAL

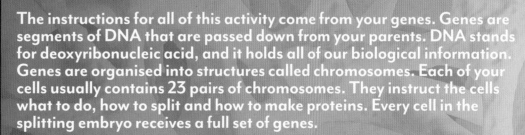

The instructions for all of this activity come from your genes. Genes are segments of DNA that are passed down from your parents. DNA stands for deoxyribonucleic acid, and it holds all of our biological information. Genes are organised into structures called chromosomes. Each of your cells usually contains 23 pairs of chromosomes. They instruct the cells what to do, how to split and how to make proteins. Every cell in the splitting embryo receives a full set of genes.

HORMONAL SYSTEM

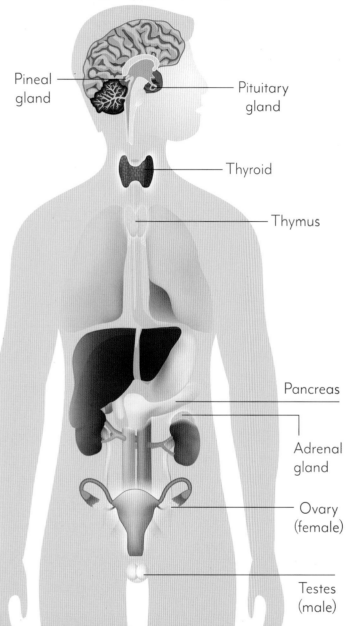

Pineal gland

Pituitary gland

Thyroid

Thymus

Pancreas

Adrenal gland

Ovary (female)

Testes (male)

FUNCTION:
Hormone regulation

MAIN STRUCTURES:
Endocrine glands and hormones

WORKS CLOSELY WITH:
The nervous and immune systems

MEDICAL FIELD:
Endocrinology ("end-o-krin-olo-gee")

Hormones control growth, emotions, digestion and healing, among other things. You can think of hormones as chemical messages. They're sent through the body by endocrine glands, the biggest of which can be found in the brain. The pituitary gland, at the bottom of the brain, controls how much of each hormone is produced by other glands. It also emits some growth and urinary hormones. The hypothalamus, about the size of an almond, monitors temperature and sensations of hunger, thirst and tiredness. Outside the brain, other glands, including the pancreas, thyroid and adrenal glands, control things such as how quickly cells carry out their jobs, and manage sugar levels in the bloodstream.

PUBERTY BLUES

Boys and girls have different reproductive organs, and some of those organs are involved in the hormonal system. Boys have testes and girls have ovaries. They each produce different hormones, which influence changes in our bodies during **puberty**.

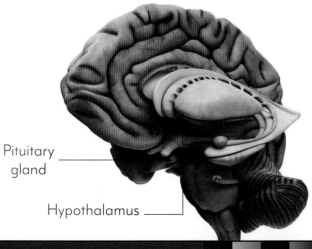

Pituitary gland

Hypothalamus

Designua/SS; valterZ/SS; Axel_Kock/SS; SciePro/SS.

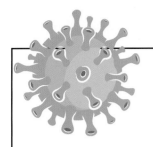

IMMUNE SYSTEM

SAFETY NETWORK

Many different organs and tissues uniquely contribute to the immune system. The spleen creates new immune cells, removes abnormal cells and filters the blood. The appendix uses immune cells to protect good bacteria. The lymphatic network drains a fluid called lymph from tissues, filtering bacteria and moving white blood cells around. This network includes the adenoids, tonsils, thymus, Peyer's patches and bone marrow.

FUNCTION: Defends against disease

MAIN STRUCTURES: Blood, lymph and lymph glands

WORKS CLOSELY WITH: The cardiovascular system

MEDICAL FIELD: Immunology ("im-mu-nol-o-gee")

The immune system defends the body against disease. It works hard to keep bacteria, viruses, parasites and fungi out of the body so you don't get sick. If anything does invade your body, the cells of your immune system will try to destroy it. The white blood cells that travel around our bloodstream are our immune cells. There are seven types: neutrophils, which target bacteria and fungi; eosinophils, which look for large parasites; basophils, which trigger allergic responses; monocytes, which clean up dead cells; mast cells, which provide general protection, t-cells, which fight viruses and cancers; and b-cells, which memorise how to make proteins that attack foreign **microbes**.

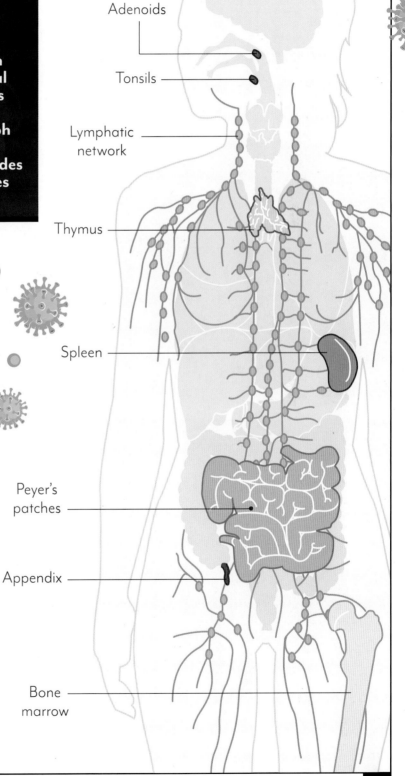

Adenoids

Tonsils

Lymphatic network

Thymus

Spleen

Peyer's patches

Appendix

Bone marrow

HOW DOES THE BODY MOVE?

You think it, and your body does it – but there's more involved than just thinking!

When you make the decision to move, your brain sends an electrical message through the nervous system to the muscles in that part of your body. It will command that muscle, or a group of muscles, to contract or expand. A muscle is a big woven group of fibres, so it is capable of doing both. Where bones meet at joints like your elbow, a system of pulleys and cords allow your body to bend. These are tendons and ligaments, strong fibres of **collagen** that link bones and muscles. When muscles contract, they can pull bones by pulling on tendons, but the same muscle can't pull the bone back. Our muscles work in pairs of flexors and extensors – the flexor will contract to bend a joint, and the extensor will contract to straighten it back out. You have hinge joints in your knees and elbows, pivot joints in your neck and forearms, gliding joints in your ankles, wrists and backbone, a saddle joint in your thumb, and ball and socket joints in your shoulders and hips.

HANDY SKILLS

In your hand, for instance, the muscles that are responsible for moving your fingers are in your palm and forearm. They move tendons that link to the small bones of your hands – when you bend your fingers back and forth, you can see them moving in your wrist and in the back of your hand.

Abdominal muscles help maintain good posture as you run, which aids in preventing injury.

The quadriceps at the front and the hamstrings at the back of the thighs help to straighten and bend the knee.

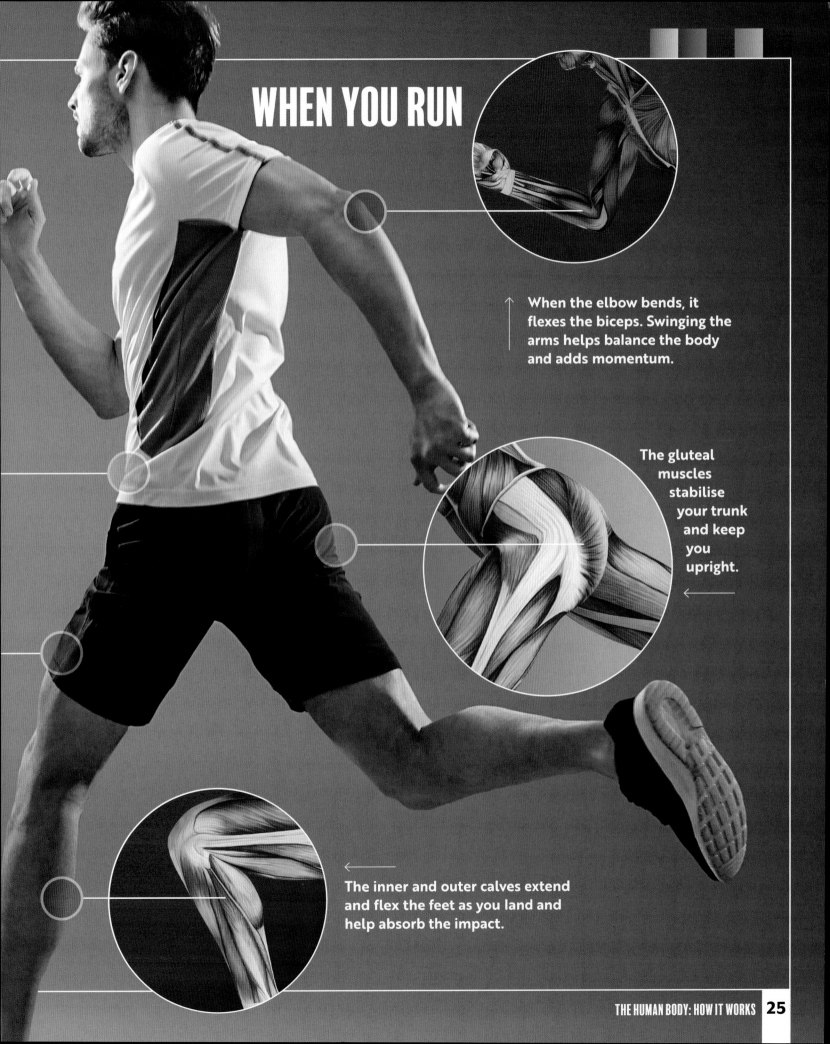

WHEN YOU RUN

When the elbow bends, it flexes the biceps. Swinging the arms helps balance the body and adds momentum.

The gluteal muscles stabilise your trunk and keep you upright.

The inner and outer calves extend and flex the feet as you land and help absorb the impact.

URINARY SYSTEM

FUNCTION:
Eliminates liquid waste

MAIN STRUCTURES:
Kidneys, bladder and urethra

WORKS CLOSELY WITH:
The cardiovascular system

MEDICAL FIELD:
Urology ("u-ro-lo-gee")

Before blood returns to the heart and lungs to be re-oxygenated, it passes through the kidneys. Blood comes in through the renal artery and into the kidneys, underneath the ribs on either side of the back, organs which help the body to filter out waste. A high-pressure system squeezes out the waste, along with watery parts of the blood, turning it into urine. Clean blood is sent back through the renal vein. Every minute, about one litre of blood passes through the kidneys. It takes the kidneys about 50 minutes to filter all of the blood in the body, and it continues the cycle over and over.

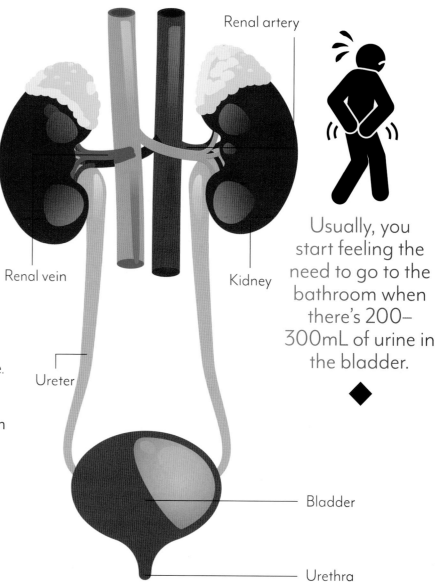

Renal artery

Renal vein

Kidney

Ureter

Bladder

Urethra

Usually, you start feeling the need to go to the bathroom when there's 200–300mL of urine in the bladder.

◆

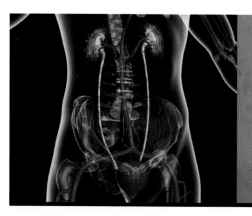

A FULL BLADDER

Inside each kidney there is around a million filtering units called nephrons. Nephrons remove any sugars, proteins, minerals or salts from the urine. It then flows down the ureter to the bladder, a stretchy organ that holds the urine until it reaches a high enough level for the nervous system to tell the brain it's time to go to the bathroom. A healthy adult produces about 1–2L of urine each day.

VectorMine/SS; Mr. Rashad/SS; Anton Nalivayko/SS; Pretty Vectors/SS; Naeblys/SS; sciencepics/SS.

INTEGUMENTARY SYSTEM

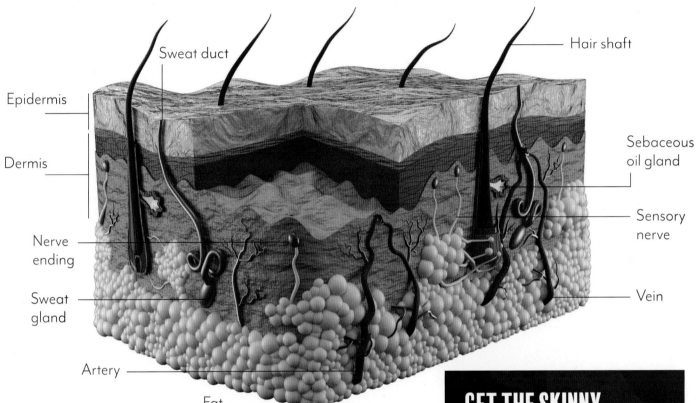

Sweat duct

Epidermis

Dermis

Nerve ending

Sweat gland

Artery

Fat

Hair shaft

Sebaceous oil gland

Sensory nerve

Vein

FUNCTION:
Protection

MAIN STRUCTURES:
Skin, hair and nails

WORKS CLOSELY WITH:
The nervous system

MEDICAL FIELD:
Dermatology ("der-mat-olo-gee")

The cells of your epidermis completely regrow in a month.

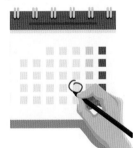

The integumentary system is the most visible body system – it's made up of the skin, hair and nails. Skin protects the body from damage, helps the body to stay the right temperature, and works with the nervous system to give us the sense of touch. Hair helps protect us too. On the head, it prevents sun damage, the eyelashes stop sweat and other small particles from getting into the eyes, and the fine hairs in the nose and ears filter out dust from the air.

GET THE SKINNY

The skin is made up of two major layers: the epidermis, which is the outermost layer, and the dermis. The epidermis is made up of **epithelial** cells, and millions of dead epithelial cells fall off you every day. The dermis is made up of connective tissues which makes your skin elastic. Inside the dermis are sweat glands. These glands help us to control our body temperature by **secreting** water to the surface through the pores in our skin, or along tiny hair follicles.

WHY DO WE GET SICK?

Our bodies can break down in many different ways.

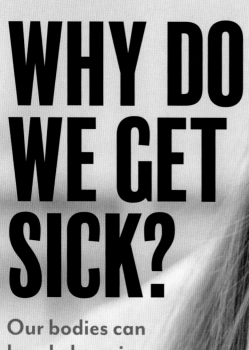

Sometimes we get sick with infectious or non-infectious diseases. Maybe we break a bone or our body simply stops working the way it should as we get older.

Infectious diseases are caused by pathogens entering our body. Pathogens are things like bacteria and viruses, and they can enter our body when we breathe or eat, or through openings in our skin. These cause an infection, which damages cells in our body.

Viruses are small organisms that replicate themselves inside our cells, and this includes ailments such as chickenpox, ebola, influenza and measles. COVID-19 is a highly infectious viral disease caused by a new strain of coronavirus. The disease spread across the entire world in 2020, giving rise to the worst **pandemic** in over 100 years. By April 2021, more than 128 million people worldwide had been diagnosed with COVID-19, resulting in nearly 3 million deaths.

Ermolaev Alexander/SS, Vadym Zaitsev/SS, Kateryna Kon/SS.

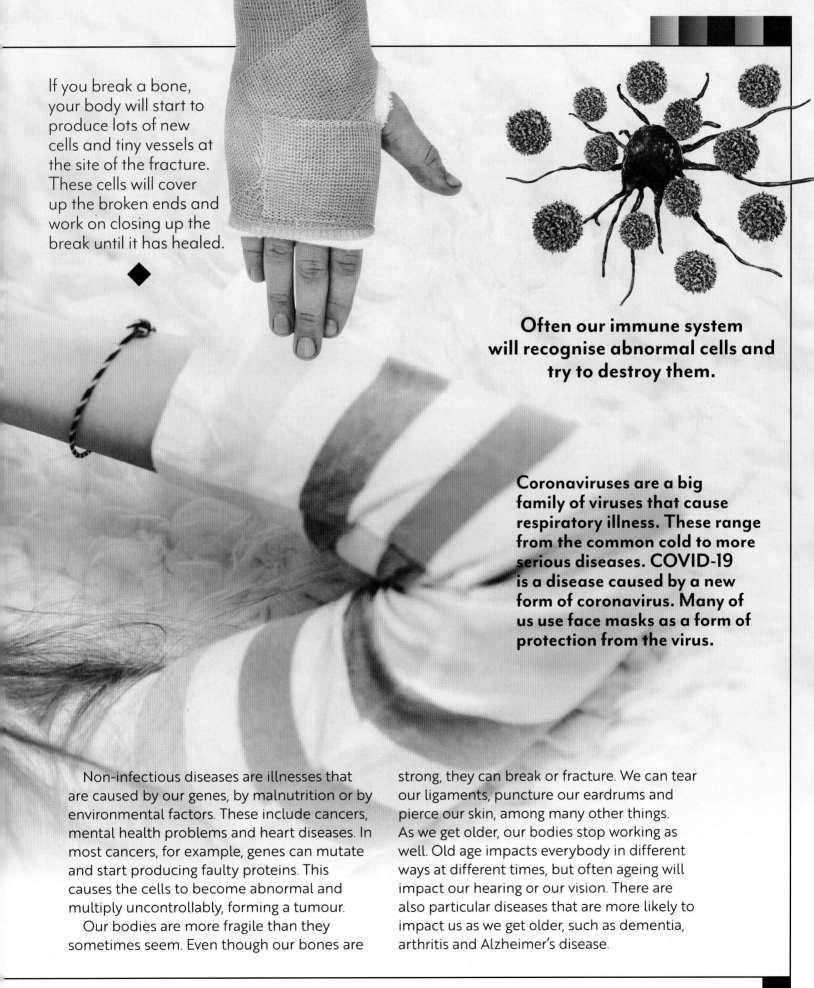

If you break a bone, your body will start to produce lots of new cells and tiny vessels at the site of the fracture. These cells will cover up the broken ends and work on closing up the break until it has healed.

Often our immune system will recognise abnormal cells and try to destroy them.

Coronaviruses are a big family of viruses that cause respiratory illness. These range from the common cold to more serious diseases. COVID-19 is a disease caused by a new form of coronavirus. Many of us use face masks as a form of protection from the virus.

Non-infectious diseases are illnesses that are caused by our genes, by malnutrition or by environmental factors. These include cancers, mental health problems and heart diseases. In most cancers, for example, genes can mutate and start producing faulty proteins. This causes the cells to become abnormal and multiply uncontrollably, forming a tumour.

Our bodies are more fragile than they sometimes seem. Even though our bones are strong, they can break or fracture. We can tear our ligaments, puncture our eardrums and pierce our skin, among many other things. As we get older, our bodies stop working as well. Old age impacts everybody in different ways at different times, but often ageing will impact our hearing or our vision. There are also particular diseases that are more likely to impact us as we get older, such as dementia, arthritis and Alzheimer's disease.

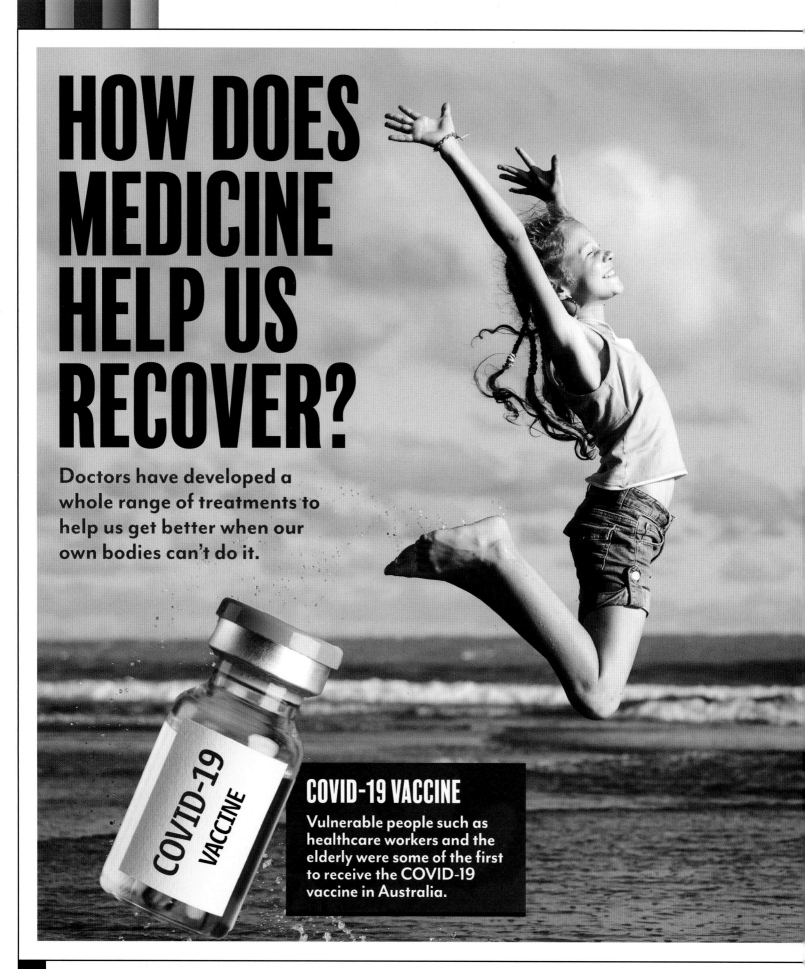

HOW DOES MEDICINE HELP US RECOVER?

Doctors have developed a whole range of treatments to help us get better when our own bodies can't do it.

COVID-19 VACCINE

COVID-19 VACCINE

Vulnerable people such as healthcare workers and the elderly were some of the first to receive the COVID-19 vaccine in Australia.

Therapy is the treatment of a medical problem and may include medicine or surgery. It also includes treatments such as physical therapy for our muscles and bones, counselling for our mental health, nutrition, and many other kinds of help. If you see a doctor, they may recommend you seek the treatment of a specialised therapist with expertise in that particular area.

Sometimes the body can't or doesn't produce enough of a certain chemical. People with diabetes, for example, can't produce enough insulin to reliably regulate the sugar levels in their bloodstream. A doctor will teach them how to monitor their sugar levels and provide them with **synthetic** insulin that they can inject to adjust it to a healthy level.

Vaccines are preventive treatments and are the most effective method for stopping the spread of infectious diseases. A vaccine usually contains an agent that will stimulate the immune system into recognising a type of pathogen and destroying it. The immune system will remember the type of pathogen so, should you encounter the real version, the body remembers how to fight it. People are regularly vaccinated against diseases such as chickenpox, diphtheria, rubella, mumps, measles, polio and hepatitis A and B. The development of these vaccines has dramatically changed the rates of infection. For example, in 1988 there were some 350,000 cases of polio recorded around the world. In 2020, there was only 140. Researchers have successfully developed a number of different vaccines to combat the spread of COVID-19. By March 2021, over 458

MODERN MEDICINE

Antibiotics are a type of drug used to treat bacterial infections. Along with vaccinations, the development of antibiotics revolutionised medicine. They kill or inhibit the growth of bacteria and have helped lead to the near eradication of diseases that were once widespread, such as tuberculosis.

million vaccine doses were administered across 73 countries, becoming the biggest vaccination campaign in human history.

Pain relievers, also known as analgesics, are a type of drug that targets your nervous system to reduce the sensation of pain, as well as reducing **inflammation**. There are various types of painkillers, including paracetamol, codeine, aspirin and ibuprofen. These all work slightly differently. Many people take pain relievers while they are healing or recovering, or to manage long-term pain symptoms.

Surgical treatments have been practised by humans for thousands of years. There's archaeological evidence that trepanning, a surgical operation in which a hole is drilled into the head to relieve pressure on the brain, was taking place in 6500BC. Since then, surgery has advanced dramatically; and is now used to treat a variety of conditions. You can have artificial devices like pacemakers implanted, tissues removed, organs transplanted, and many other surgical treatments. These days, we even have robotic surgery, which ensures more precise, safer and faster operations.

Antibiotics actually cause the cell walls of bacteria to burst!

GLOSSARY

Auditory: Relating to the sense of hearing.

Carbohydrates: Molecules that aid in energy transportation around the body, including glucose and lactose.

Cognitive: Concerned with the act of perceiving, knowing and other mental processes.

Collagen: A protein that holds the body together.

Embryo: An unborn baby in the process of development.

Enzymes: Protein that provoke a chemical reaction.

Epithelial: Tissues of the skin.

Fascia: A band of tissue that surrounds organs and muscles, keeping their shape.

Inflammation: When part of the body becomes reddened, hot, and painful, in reaction to infection or injury.

Microbes: Tiny organisms.

Olfactory: Relating to the sense of smell.

Ossicles: Very small bones.

Pandemic: The worldwide spread of a disease.

Proteins: Substances formed by amino acids, found in all cells.

Puberty: The process of developing from a child into an adult.

Spatial: Relating to or occupying space.

Synthetic: Created in a laboratory.

Transfusion: A transfer of donated blood into another person's circulatory system.

Villi: Small structures in the small intestine that help to absorb digested food.

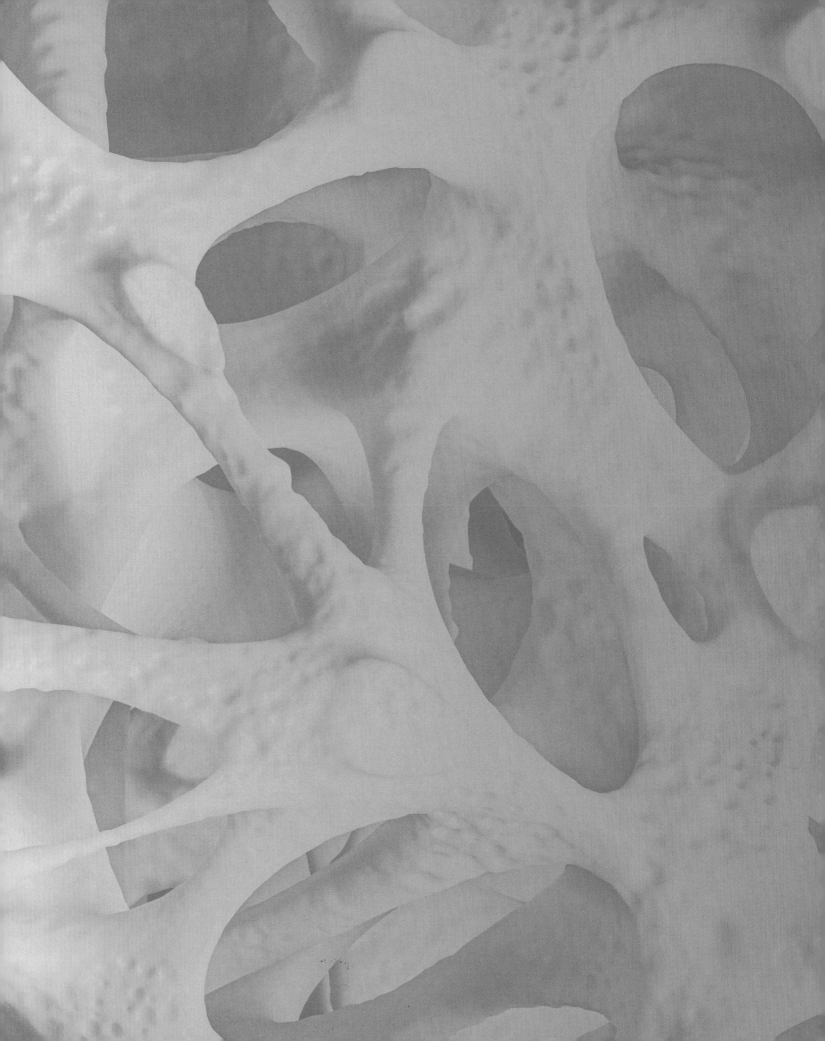